Ketogenic Diet

30 Day Ketogenic Diet Plan

LELA GIBSON

CONTENTS

KETOGENIC DIET

Introduction

I want to thank you and congratulate you for buying the book, *"Ketogenic Diet: 30 Day Ketogenic Diet Plan"*.

This book has an easy to follow 30 day Ketogenic diet plan that you can use to lose weight effortlessly.

If you are overweight, you know just how frustrating it can get to try to lose weight only to fail repeatedly while at it. What is even more frustrating is that most people think that those who are overweight or obese are like that because they don't put as much effort to losing weight. If only they knew how much effort we have to put in even when we don't make visible progress, they wouldn't be so insensitive!

But as you are well aware, people won't stop talking and making suggestions on what you can do to lose weight and keep it off. You too won't stop thinking and feeling that your weight could be increasing your odds of developing various health complications. That's not all; you won't stop feeling that you really should do something about your excess weight to be fitter, leaner, healthier, to fit in certain clothes, to look better etc.

What then can you do to actually make your goal of losing weight and keeping it off a reality? Well, I know you've already tried many things unsuccessfully. Have you heard about the Ketogenic diet? Since you are reading this book, it is likely that you've heard great things about the diet including the fact that it might be the secret to you losing weight and keeping it off.

Are you now looking for information to make the diet part of your life? Lucky for you, this book has comprehensive information on how to follow a 30-day plan to losing weight and keeping it off with the Ketogenic diet. The book provides a brief background of the Ketogenic diet, the benefits that you stand to get from the diet as well as a 30-day plan, with recipes, to help you realize your goal of losing weight and keeping it off.

PS: Even if you are new to the Ketogenic diet, you will find this book helpful as it will help you to realize effortless weight loss. Don't worry; the Ketogenic diet is backed by science so you can be sure that whatever you will be doing has been scientifically proven!

Let's begin.

Thanks again for buying this book. I hope you enjoy it!

An Introduction To The Ketogenic Diet

What Is It?

The ketogenic is a special diet mainly focused on weight loss and maintenance of general body health. It is inherently composed of high amount of fats, low carbohydrates and medium proteins. What's the purpose of all this? Well, the purpose of pairing low carbohydrates intake with high fat and moderate protein intake is to push the body to a nutritional state referred to as ketosis. This is what makes it to be referred to as Ketogenic diet- without ketosis, you cannot be said to be in a Ketogenic diet.

How does it bring about ketosis, you might ask? Well, by reducing the amount of carbohydrates that you take greatly, you end up forcing the body to start metabolizing stored body fat, which, when metabolized leads to the production of ketone bodies. Let me explain this:

The diet is based on a simple principle that to lose weight and improve our mental and physical health, we have to, among other things, reduce fat production and storage in the body and achieve a particular state known as ketosis. The diet is actually meant to help your body burn fats for fuel instead of carbohydrates.

This is what I mean:

As an average person under normal circumstances, your body burns carbohydrates (which generally take the largest share of a regular American meal since we follow USDAs food pyramid, which has carbs at the bottom of the pyramid) for energy. This occurs when your body converts these carbohydrates into glucose, which is then either used for energy directly or converted to glycogen and then stored in the liver and muscle cells to be used in future. This process takes place with the help of insulin hormone, which is produced by the beta cells of the pancreas. Insulin usually tells the cells to open up so as to take up glucose since the cells don't have their own inbuilt mechanism of absorbing glucose. Insulin keeps the 'doors' to the cells open to allow them to take as much glucose as possible i.e. until they have had enough. If the available glucose in the bloodstream is more than what the cells can use, the excess is channeled to the liver where it is converted to glycogen, which is then stored in the liver and muscle cells.

The problem comes when these stores are full (yes, the glycogen stores can only take about 2000kcal of energy at a time) and you experience some sort of 'spill over' and the excess is converted into fatty acids and glycerol, which is then transported in the bloodstream to the fat stores around the body. The depositing of fatty acids and glycerol (in the form of triglycerides) is what causes weight gain if it takes place over time. This therefore means that we accumulate fat not because of eating fat but carbohydrates (especially the simple carbs, which are easily broken down and processed by the body).

The ketogenic diet seeks to minimize your intake of carbohydrates as much as possible (to a point where the body barely has enough carbohydrates to fuel various body processes) so that your body is forced to turn to the next available source of fuel in the body, which is fat because things have to keep ticking anyway. On the Ketogenic diet, you only take a moderate amount of proteins i.e. enough for muscle repair and maintenance- not more.

When your carb intake is low the reverse of the above explanation happens. For starters, with reduced carbohydrates intake, glucose levels reduce and this in turn leads to reduced insulin production. As the levels of insulin reduce due to reducing levels of dietary glucose in the bloodstream, the pancreas releases glucagon hormone from the alpha cells. The role of glucagon is to trigger the liver to break down glycogen into glucose, which is then used up for energy, just like dietary glucose. But since glycogen stores have a limited capacity, the stores soon start running out. In such a situation (absence of carbs/glucose), the fat cells start releasing triglycerides into the bloodstream where they (triglycerides) are transported to the liver for breakdown. When they get to the liver, they are broken down into their constituent components i.e. fatty acids and glycerol after which the former is broken down further in a process known as ketogenesis to produce a ketone body known as acetoacetate. Acetoacetate is then broken down into two more types of ketones: Beta-hydroxybutyrate (BHB) and Acetone.

These ketones are used by the entire body as fuel including the brain. The lower the amount of carbs that you take, the more ketones you produce. You are said to be in optimal ketosis when your blood ketone readings range between 1.5 – 3 mmol/L. At that time, you at an optimal fat burning rate.

If this goes on for a while, it brings about weight loss (because of several reasons) along with other benefits that we will discuss in the next chapter.

How the keto diet brings about weight loss:

1: It results to the production of ketones, which have appetite suppression properties

2: Fat itself is filling and has appetite suppression properties, which means that by eating more fat, you reduce the urge to eat and ultimately end up taking less food

3: When you metabolize glycogen, you end up losing a lot of water weight- 1g of glycogen takes 4g of water to store so as you use up glycogen, you end up shedding lots of water weight.

4: Reducing carb intake forces your body to start using fats for energy, which ultimately results to ketone production and subsequent weight loss

5: The low carb foods allowed in the diet e.g. veggies are filling and low in calories, which ultimately means you get filled with fewer carb. This ultimately helps you lose weight fast.

Note: I know you might be wondering; so what's the point of eating more fats on a keto diet? Well, the main reason is to help shift the body's metabolism from carb metabolism to fat metabolism. In simpler terms, it helps put the body in a fat burning mode, which ultimately helps to burn body fat. While you are required to take lots of fat, it doesn't mean you are free to take an unlimited amount of fat; you should aim to create a calorie deficit of at least 500 calories per day (based on your daily calorie requirement) to bring about weight loss of at least 1 pound per week.

So which benefits should you expect by following the keto diet besides weight loss, which we've already discussed how it happens? Let's discuss that next.

What Should You Expect From The Keto Diet?

1: They improve your brain's health

The processing of ketones is associated with hormones and enzymes that are different from those associated with glucose metabolism. This causes a cascade of effects that work towards improving your brain health. I will briefly go over two of the main ways ketone bodies improve your brain.

-They act as neuroprotective antioxidants and provide better energy

First of all, ketones basically act as antioxidants. This way, they prevent harmful oxygen species from causing damage to the cells in your brain. At the same time, ketones are typically more efficient as energy sources per unit oxygen than sugar. This means that if you want to maintain the health of your aging brain cells, burning ketones may come in handy in maintaining the health of such cells because over time, they (the cells) easily become unable to efficiently use glucose as fuel.

That's not all; the ketones also increase the efficiency and production of mitochondria. The diet itself brings about a synchronized upregulation (increasing the response to stimulus) of the genes associated with the mitochondria and the genes involved in the metabolism of energy while stimulating the synthesis of mitochondria themselves. This in overall improves the performance of the brain cells and protects them from Parkinson's disease, Alzheimer's disease among other neurodegenerative diseases, and stroke.

-Increase the levels of GABA and Glutamate

Glutamate is the main excitatory neurotransmitter of the brain. It gives rise to GABA, which is the main inhibitory neurotransmitter of the brain. Glutamate is basically important for memory, neural communication, regulation and learning. However, when glutamate is stimulated excessively, it usually causes damage and death to nerve cells- when this occurs, you start seeing issues such as ALS (amyotrophic lateral sclerosis), Alzheimer's disease, multiple sclerosis and Parkinson's disease starting to develop. Even though the mechanisms are not very clear, ketones tend to reduce the levels of glutamate and increase GABA to assist prevent cell damage in the brain and improve their overall function. This is because GABA counteracts the action of glutamate in the nerve cells to maintain a good balance in the brain.

-Helps in the management of diabetes type 2

When you eat large amounts of carbs repeatedly, your blood sugar spikes and a lot of insulin is obviously needed to lower it. This results in blood sugar crashes- something medical experts call 'blood sugar rollercoaster'. With time, you may realize that more medication and insulin are required to control the highs of this roller coaster, something that usually upturns the cost of diabetic care. Logically, the solution would be getting off the blood sugar roller coaster in the first place. This is where the ketogenic diet comes in. By virtue of being a low carb diet, the keto diet stops the blood glucose crash/spike cycle and even helps you reduce or eliminate the need for medications like metformin and the need for extra insulin.

Think about it; the insulin hormone works to take the excess sugar from the blood and into the cells. With the keto diet, you are taking less carbs, thus, there's no need for a lot of insulin which your body can easily become insensitive to when produced frequently and in high amounts- this is a main problem facing patients of diabetes type 2.

-Helps in the management of cancer

The benefits of the keto diet regarding prevention and treatment of cancer are increasingly becoming clearer and widespread every day. If you are keen on this topic, you'd know that many cancer patients following a ketogenic are progressively reporting to be experiencing many benefits.

The concept here is simple. Cancer cells usually depend on sugar as their main source of fuel. Any means of systematically and steadily depriving these cells of glucose is a great way to starve cancer to its death and I can't think of a way that can do that better than a ketogenic diet.

Simple as it may seem, this concept is supported by studies such as <u>this one</u> and <u>this one</u>.

There was a feasibility <u>study</u> conducted in 2012 on ten patients of cancer, which provided very good results. The patients were put on a keto diet for 28 days and after the period, five of them stabilized, four were still progressing and one of them was seen to have had a slight improvement (the disease proliferation levels had dropped a bit).

It is worth noting that the patients in this study had attempted to incorporate all the other cancer treatment methods before, but none of them had really worked. After four weeks of following this diet, about 60 percent of them either improved or stalled.

-*The diet makes sure you stay young*

There are many HEALTHY ways of staying young and one of the surest ways is making sure the oxidative stress in your body remains low. An ideal keto diet reduces the levels of insulin and facilitates a constant supply of ketones throughout your body, which your body then uses as fuel. According to research, reducing the levels of insulin in your body consequently reduces oxidative stress (read more). Other researches scientists have also discovered how to use the keto diet when it comes to anti-aging.

A good ketogenic diet decreases insulin levels and allows for production of ketones, which your body uses as fuel. Research shows that when you reduce the levels of insulin in your body, you decrease oxidative stress.

Another study shows that a ketogenic diet decreases the oxidative damage to the body and conversely increases uric acid production among other strong antioxidants. This alone has noteworthy implications because according to recent reports which you can go through (also here) suggest that the ketone bodies that a ketogenic diet produces relieve and reverse a number of neurological disorders that oxidative stress is seen to be a cause, at the cellular level. This includes Alzheimer's disease, traumatic brain injury, ALS, stroke and Parkinson's disease. There's another study as well that linked beta-hydroxybutyrate (a ketone body) in slowing down aging by initiating a gene expression that modifies the factors related to aging.

Again, being on a ketogenic diet increases <u>mitochondrial glutathione</u>, an important antioxidant that works within the mitochondria directly to boost the mitochondrial function. This is important because the antioxidants that are normally ingested normally like the ones in our food do not reach the mitochondria easily.

Improved mitochondrial functions also means you benefit in another way- you get to experience increased levels of energy as explained below:

Boosts your levels of energy

Many studies today show that a ketogenic diet does improve the function of the mitochondria, and the levels of free radicals in the body as well (please <u>read more</u>). Mitochondria are simple but important structures found in the cells that normally give out energy by processing food and oxygen for your body to use. When these structures function better, it means your cells will naturally produce more energy and in the end, you start feeling more energetic and lively.

On the other hand, when oxygen interacts with particular molecules in your body, radicals are produced. These radicals tend to reduce the levels of energy your body produces because they essentially cause a lot of damage to the mitochondria. They tend to be very reactive and destroy these structures slowly. In the long run, they may cause cell death, after a sustained poor cell performance. Having less production of free radicals in the body means better neurological stability and a healthy function at the cellular level, which makes sure energy in the body is better utilized.

This means that all the focus of your body goes to production of more energy instead of concentrating on the repair of the energy triggered by free radicals.

You however need to note that to trigger more production of mitochondria, you have to consider combining ketogenic dieting and physical exercises because this obviously helps manage the intensified energy demands in your body.

We could go on and on about the benefits of the ketogenic diet because they are actually countless; but I'm sure you are already curious about what this diet entails. Next, we will discuss what you should eat while on the diet to bring about the above benefits and much more.

The Ketogenic Diet: What To Eat

Since we're close to the best part, I'll just go straight to the point here.

Fats

When it comes to fats, stick to the following list:

Saturated fats

- Cheese

- Lard and cream

- Poultry with skin

- Lamb

- Whole-fat milk or reduced dairy products

- Butter

- Beef fat tallow

- Fatty beef

Monounsaturated fats

- Nuts and seeds

- Peanut butter

- Avocados

- Safflower oil and

- Canola oil

- Sesame oil

- Peanut oil

- Olive oil

Polyunsaturated fats

- Chia seeds

- Flaxseed

- Fish oil

- Fish

For the oils, use:

- Coconut oil

- Avocado oil

- Macadamia oil

- Olive oil

- Flaxseed oil

- MTC oil

Note: Always avoid trans-fats

Trans-fats are unsaturated forms of fats only with a different structure from that of the normal unsaturated fats. Trans-fats are discouraged because they harm the body's health, starting with the heart.

Trans-fats are typically common in the following foods:

- Stick margarine and Vegetable shortening

- Refrigerated dough products (like cinnamon rolls and biscuits)

- Grain-based desserts (like cookies, cakes, and frozen pies)

- Fast food

- Savory snacks (like microwave popcorn and crackers)

- Frostings that are 'ready to use'

- Frozen pizza

- Coffee creamer

Proteins

- Peanut butter- natural peanut butter is best

- Shell fish

  - ✓ Squid

  - ✓ Clams

  - ✓ Scallops

  - ✓ Lobster

  - ✓ Mussels

  - ✓ Oyster

  - ✓ Crab

- Fish- anything that's wild such as:

✓ Cod

✓ Halibut

✓ Catfish

✓ Flounder

✓ Tuna

✓ Mackerel

✓ Salmon

✓ Mahi-mahi

✓ Snapper

- Cured Meats such as

✓ Pepperoni

✓ Prosciutto

✓ Salami

- Sausages

- Poultry

    ✓ Chicken

    ✓ Quail

    ✓ Pheasant

    ✓ Duck

- Whole eggs- always go for the free range eggs from a local market.

- Roasts (Pork/ Lamb/Beef)

- Steak

- Deli meats (you probably need to second check nutrition because some particular brands use carb fillers)

- Ham

- Pork

  ✓ Loin

  ✓ Steaks

  ✓ Chops

- Ribs (Beef/Pork/Lamb)

- Ground beef

Just a reminder: when purchasing meats, try getting those that contain a good fat content. You should also try going for grass fed types of meats and free-range eggs so that you are sure that you're dealing with minimal steroid hormones and bacteria. In case you didn't know, grass-fed meat usually contains a great fatty acid count.

Vegetables

- Broccoli

- Onion

- Various leafy greens like

- ▪

    - ✓ Bib lettuce

    - ✓ Arugula

    - ✓ Spinach

    - ✓ Romaine

- ✓ Asparagus

- ✓ Peas

- ✓ Parsnips

- ✓ Corn

- ✓ Garlic

- ✓ Cauliflower

- ✓ Artichoke hearts

- ✓ Cabbage

- ✓ Peppers

- ✓ Yucca

✓ Brussels sprouts

✓ Squash

✓ Mushrooms

Fruits

As you may notice, the fruits in this list are few; the ketogenic diet doesn't usually accommodate many fruits because most of them typically contain a lot of sugar (fructose). In between meals, try using the following fruits as snacks:

- Lime

- Blackberry

- Olive

- Blueberry

- Raspberry

- Cranberry

- Strawberry

- Lemon

- Avocado

Try as much as possible to stick to the foods above during your meals.

Now, let's get practical.

Let's talk about the recipes and a meal plan!

The 30-Day Keto Diet Plan with Recipes

Day 1:

Breakfast:

Avocado toad in the Hole

Serves 6

Ingredients

1/4 cup Parmesan cheese

1/2 teaspoon sea salt

6 medium eggs

1/4 teaspoon black pepper

1 teaspoon garlic powder

3 pitted medium avocados

Directions

Preheat your oven to 350 degrees F.

Remove the pits from all the avocados and halve them. Scoop a third of the 'flesh' from each one of them. The idea here is creating enough space for the eggs to fit inside.

Place all the halves in a muffin tin with their (avocados) tops facing upwards.

Sprinkle all the halves gently with black pepper, garlic powder and sea salt.

Crack one egg into the avocados and then sprinkle the cheese over the egg tops.

Place in the oven and give it 12-15 minutes to bake, until the egg white is set and isn't jiggling anymore when you wobble the pan.

Nutritional information per serving: 261 Calories, Fat 20g, Protein 14g, Carbohydrates 3g

Lunch:

Easy Keto Lasagna Stuffed Portobellos

Serves 4

Ingredients

Chopped parsley to garnish if desired

1 cup sugar free marinara sauce

4 links of Italian sausage

1 cup whole milk mozzarella cheese, shredded

1 cup whole milk ricotta cheese

4 large portobello mushrooms

Directions

Take a dry paper towel and brush off any dirt off from the mushrooms. If the mushrooms have stems, get them out then get a spoon and scrape out all the brown ribs.

Preheat oven to 375 degrees F.

Get the sausage out from the casing and press into four patties. Press every single patty into every single mushroom cap and make sure to do that all the way to the edges and sides.

Spoon a quarter cup of the ricotta into the mushroom caps and press to the edges properly; leave a dip at the center to hold the sauce.

Spoon the marinara into the mushrooms (a quarter cup for each mushroom) on top of the layer of ricotta.

Sprinkle a quarter cup of the shredded mozzarella cheese on top of each mushroom.

Place it in the oven and let it bake for 40 minutes.

You can now garnish with parsley.

Serve hot.

Save some for dinner.

Nutritional information per serving: Calories 482, Fat 36g, Protein 28g, Carbohydrates 6.5g

Dinner:

Easy Keto Lasagna Stuffed Portobellos

Day 2
Breakfast:

Cream Cheese Pancakes

Serves 4

Ingredients

2 ounces cream cheese

1 teaspoon granulated sugar substitute

2 eggs

1/2 teaspoon cinnamon

Directions

Put all the above ingredients in a blender and blend.

Give the mixture two minutes to allow the bubbles to settle.

Grease a pan with pam spray or butter and then pour in a quarter of the batter.

Leave it to cook for two minutes- you can let it turn golden, flip and cook for a minute on the other side.

Repeat all the steps with the remaining batter.

Enjoy with some berries and sugar free syrup.

Nutritional information per serving: Calories 344, Fat 29g, Protein 17g Carbohydrates 3g

Lunch:

Mocha Chia Pudding

Serves 2

Ingredients

2 tablespoons herbal coffee

1/3 cup coconut cream, undiluted

1 tablespoon Swerve

2 tablespoons Cacao nibs

1/3 cup dry chia seeds

1 tablespoon organic vanilla extract

Directions

Prepare a strong herbal coffee, simmering two cups of water with three tablespoons of a complete herbal blend.

After straining the coffee, blend it in vanilla extract and coconut cream, and then swerve.

Now add the cacao nibs and the chia seeds and stir them together properly.

Place them in serving containers and leave them for 30 minutes before serving.

You can now add a bit more herbal coffee to the pudding while serving and decorate by sprinkling some cacao nibs over.

Nutritional information per serving: Calories: 257, Fat 20.25g, Protein 7g, Carbs 2.25g

Dinner:

Low Carb Shepherd's Pie

Serves 6

Ingredients

1/4 cup grated parmesan

1 cup heavy cream

1 cup tomatoes (chopped)

1 lb. ground beef, lamb or turkey

1 teaspoon dried thyme

1 cup shredded cheese

3 minced garlic cloves

2 12 ounce packages of cooked & well drained riced cauliflower

1/2 cup celery (chopped)

1/4 cup yellow onion (chopped)

1/4 cup oil

Directions

Add the oil to a large skillet and heat it.

Now add the celery, onions, ground meat and garlic and fry until the meat turns brown.

Turn off the heat and then stir the tomatoes in quickly; place this mixture into a casserole dish measuring 10x7 inches

Blend the cauliflower, thyme, cream and the cheeses until you've got a mixture resembling mashed potatoes more than riced cauliflower.

Add the cauliflower evenly over the meat in the dish and leave it to bake for about 35 minutes at 350 degrees.

After cooling, cut and serve.

Save some for tomorrow's lunch.

Nutritional information per serving: Calories 469, Fat 39g, Protein 23g, Carbohydrates 6g

Day 3
Breakfast:

Almond Cream Cheese Pancakes

Serves 4

Ingredients

Butter, for frying

1 teaspoon erythritol (optional)

1/2 teaspoon cinnamon

4 eggs

125g or 1/2 cup full fat cream cheese

60g or 1/2 cup and an extra 1-tablespoon almond flour

Directions

Add all the ingredients in a blender and blend.

Melt butter in a non-stick pan and fry the pancakes. Turn once over when the center starts bubbling. The pancakes should be about 10-12 centimeters in diameter- just about the proper size to fit them in a toaster the following day in case you are lucky to have any left overs.

Nutritional information per serving

Calories 234.8, Fats 19.9g, Proteins 11.2g, Carbohydrates 3.9g

Lunch:

Low carb shepherd's pie

Dinner:

Low Carb Italian Eggs in Purgatory

Serves 5

Ingredients:

5 precooked and chopped small breakfast sausage links

1/4 cup minced onion

2 peeled and minced cloves of garlic

2 fresh basil leaves that are torn into small pieces

1/8 teaspoon dried oregano

1/4 teaspoon pepper

1 tablespoon Italian parsley, chopped *optional

1/2 cup diced zucchini

1/3 cup red bell pepper, diced

1 ½ cup of tomato sauce or puree

1 tablespoon olive oil

1/4 teaspoon sea salt

5 eggs

1 tablespoon Parmesan (optional), omit for paleo

Directions

Get a large and deep skillet, add olive oil and heat.

Add the garlic, onions and bell peppers. Cook while stirring until the onions become translucent- this should take about five minutes.

Add the chopped sausages and zucchini then stir and cook until the zucchini become soft- this should take about 4 minutes.

Now add pepper, oregano, tomato sauce, salt and basil. Stir and keep heating for 3-5 minutes until the sauce is bubbling and reducing a bit.

Create a hole in the sauce using a spoon on the outer pan edges. Make one in the middle section and four on the outer edges.

Crack the eggs into the wells- one for each well.

Cover the pan and reduce the heat to low; simmer for 8-12 minutes, or until the eggs cook as you desire.

You can now top with parsley and parmesan.

Serve and enjoy!

Save some for tomorrow's lunch.

Nutritional information per serving: Calories 219, Fats 16g, Proteins 9g, Carbohydrates- 5g

Day 4
Breakfast:

Green Smoothie Bowl

Serves 1

Ingredients

For the green smoothie bowl

2 tablespoon lemon juice

1/4 cup ice cubes

1/4 cup Erythritol, or any other sweetener - to taste

3/4 cup of unsweetened coconut milk

1/2 medium avocados

1 cup Spinach

1/2 scoop Perfect Keto MCT Oil Powder

1/2 scoop Perfect Keto Collagen

For the toppings

1 teaspoon Hemp seeds

1/2 teaspoon Chia seeds

1 teaspoon Coconut flakes

Desired berries (optional)

Directions

Puree the avocado, collagen, MCT oil powder, coconut milk, erythritol ice, lemon juice and ice cubes in a powerful blender until very smooth.

Pour the smoothie into a bowl and top with chia seeds, coconut flakes and hemp seeds.

You can now add berries of your choice if you want.

Nutritional information per serving: Calories 319, Fat-26g, Protein-10g, Carbohydrates-15g

Lunch:

Low Carb Italian Eggs in Purgatory

Dinner:

Easy Leftover Turkey Casserole Recipe With Mayonnaise

Serves 10 (1 cup each)

Ingredients

3 cups turkey (cooked, shredded or cubed)

4cups green beans (cooked and salted lightly)

1 1/2 cups of sugar-free cranberry sauce

1 cup shredded Cheddar cheese

2 cloves minced garlic

1/2 cup Mayonnaise or Greek yogurt

1/2 cup crumbled goat cheese

1/2 cup chopped Walnuts (optional)

Directions

Preheat your oven to 350 degrees F.

Then line your dish with a foil if it's not glass or stoneware.

Stir together the green beans, shredded cheddar cheese, minced garlic, mayonnaise and turkey in a large bowl and spread evenly in the casserole dish.

Spread the sauce properly over the casserole and top with walnuts and goat cheese.

Let it bake for 20-30 minutes until the casserole becomes hot and the edges bubbly.

Nutritional information per serving: Calories: 244, Fat 17g, Total Carbohydrates 9g, Protein 13g

Day 5
Breakfast:

Avocado toad in the Hole

Lunch:

Keto Lasagna with Zucchini Noodles

Serves 4

Ingredients

16 ounces ground beef

1 zucchini large

1 cup Rao's marinara sauce

4 ounces mozzarella cheese shredded

Directions

Preheat your oven to 350 degrees F and then peel the zucchini into strips; leave out the seedy core. Now salt it and leave it to sit for 15 minutes; blot with some paper towels.

Brown the ground beef in a pan then add marinara and season well with pepper and salt.

Layer it into a little casserole dish with mozzarella at the bottom, then ricotta, zucchini, meat, ricotta, zucchini, meat.

Cover it with a foil and bake for 30 minutes. Uncover it and broil for about three minutes so that it browns at the top.

Enjoy!

Save some for dinner.

Nutritional information per serving: Calories: 544, Fat 41g, Protein 34g, Carbohydrates 6g

Dinner:

Keto Lasagna with Zucchini Noodles

Day 6
Breakfast:

Cream Cheese Pancakes

Lunch:

Mocha Chia Pudding

Dinner:

Easy Shrimp Avocado Salad With Tomatoes And Feta

Serves 2

Ingredients

8 ounces shrimp peeled, deveined and patted dry

1 small beefsteak tomato drained and diced

1/3 cup freshly chopped parsley or cilantro

1 tablespoon lemon juice

1/4 teaspoon salt

1 large avocado diced

1/3 cup crumbled feta cheese

2 tablespoons salted butter, melted

1 tablespoon olive oil

1/4 teaspoon black pepper

Directions

Toss the shrimp in a bowl with melted butter until well coated.

Heat the pan for a few minutes over medium high heat until it gets hot. Now add shrimp in one layer to the pan and sear until it starts becoming pink around the edges, which should take one minute; flip the shrimp and then cook until they cook through- this should take less than one minute.

Now take the shrimp to a plate as they complete cooking and leave them to cool; meanwhile, prepare the other ingredients.

Add the diced tomato, diced avocado, lemon juice, feta cheese, cilantro, pepper, olive oil and salt to a large bowl then toss to mix.

Now add the shrimp and stir properly to mix together; you can also add more pepper and salt to taste.

Save some for tomorrow's lunch.

Nutritional information per serving: Calories 430, Fats 33g, Protein 24g, Carbohydrates 6.5g

Day 7
Breakfast:

Easy Keto Egg Salad

Serves 2

Ingredients

1 avocado, medium

1/3 Cup Mayonnaise

Splash of lemon juice (this will protect the avocado from browning)

1/2 tablespoon fresh chopped parsley

6 eggs

1 teaspoon Dijon mustard

1/8 teaspoon dill

Salt and pepper, to taste

Directions

Place the eggs in a sauce pan and cover them with water. Let them boil, turn off the heat and rest in the hot water for 10-15 minutes- could be more or less depending on what you like.

Next, run under cold water and then peel the shells.

Chop the eggs into little pieces, sprinkle with pepper and salt and set aside

Mash the avocado and sprinkle with pepper and salt.

Mix the mayo, mashed avocado, eggs, lemon juice, mustard and herbs of your preference.

Cool and serve.

Nutritional information per serving: Calories: 575, Fat 51g, Carbohydrates 2g, Protein 20g

Lunch:

Low Carb Italian Eggs in Purgatory

Dinner:

Keto Sausage and Egg Breakfast Sandwich

Serves 1

Ingredients

1 tablespoon butter

1 tablespoon mayonnaise

2 slices sharp cheddar cheese

2 large eggs

2 sausage patties, cooked

A few slices of avocado

Directions

In a large skillet, heat the butter over medium high heat and place silicone egg molds or lightly oiled mason jar rings into the pan.

Crack two eggs into the rings then whisk gently using a fork. Cover and cook for 3-4 minutes, or until the eggs have cooked through- now remove the eggs from the rings. Now remove the eggs from the rings and place one of them (eggs) on a plate. Top it with mayonnaise and top it with a sausage patty.

Top the sausage with avocado and a slice of cheese.

Place the other sausage patty on top of the avocado and use the rest of the cheese to top. Spread the rest of the mayonnaise on the second cooked egg and place it over the cheese.

Spread the rest of the mayonnaise on the other cooked egg and place it over the cheese.

Serve immediately and enjoy

Leave some for tomorrow's lunch.

Nutritional information per serving: Calories: 880, Fat 82g, Protein 32g, Carbs 6g

Day 8
Breakfast:

Almond Cream Cheese Pancakes

Lunch:

Low Carb Quiche

Serves 2 (quiches)

Ingredients

Almond Flour Crust

3/4 cup almond flour

1 large egg

2 tablespoon grated parmesan

1/4 teaspoon salt

<u>The first Quiche</u>

1 large egg

2 slices bacon (cooked)

1/2 oz. mozzarella cheese

Salt and pepper

1/2 tablespoon heavy whipping cream

4 small cherub tomatoes

1/4 teaspoon parsley

The second Quiche

2 large eggs

1 ounces frozen spinach

Salt and pepper

0.5 ounces gorgonzola cheese

1/2 tablespoon heavy whipping cream

Directions

The crust

Start by mixing all the ingredients for the crust; these include parmesan, salt, flour and egg. Combine properly until dough forms.

Split the dough into two parts and then form in the bottom/ two quiche pans. With this recipe, you should be able to make enough crust for quiche pans with a diameter of 2.4 inches.

You can make scores in dough using a knife or fork to prevent the crust from bubbling in the oven.

Leave to bake for 7 minutes at 325 degrees F. Chill.

The first Quiche

Layer mozzarella cheese, cherub tomatoes and cooked bacon at the bottom or cooled crust.

Mix the heavy whipping cream and egg and then pour onto the fillings and crust.

Season it with pepper and salt and bake for 22-25 minutes at 350 degrees F (or until cooked through fully).

The second Quiche

Layer gorgonzola and cooked thawed spinach on the cooled crust.

Mix the heavy whipping cream and two eggs and then pour the mixture over the fillings and crust. Season it with pepper and salt.

Bake until cooked through or for about 22 minutes at 350 degrees.

Enjoy!

Save some for dinner.

Nutritional information per serving: Calories: 537, Fat 44g, Protein 29g, Carbs 6g

Dinner:

Low Carb Quiche

Day 9
Breakfast:

Green Smoothie Bow

Lunch:

Crispy Pork Salad

Serves 2

Ingredients

4.58 ounces pork belly slices

0.07 ounces walnut halves

1 tablespoon stevia

¼ medium pear

½ teaspoon wholegrain mustard

2 teaspoons olive oil

2 teaspoons salt

1 teaspoon water

1.41 ounces blue cheese

½ teaspoon Dijon mustard

2 tablespoons white wine vinegar

2.12 ounces mixed greens

Directions

Set your oven to the 'broil' function.

Take the pork slices, cover them with a teaspoon of olive oil and then apply salt on both sides liberally. Now cook in the oven until it turns crispy and golden brown- this should take about 20-30 minutes.

As you wait for the pork to cook, start chopping the walnuts into smaller pieces.

Heat a pan over medium heat; add stevia and water to the pan and wait for the stevia to dissolve completely after which you'll add the chopped walnuts. Now cook for about five minutes until the liquid becomes thick and caramelized on the nuts.

Tip the nuts onto a tray to cool, but avoid touching them because they'll obviously be hot.

Chop the pear and blue vein cheese into pieces; set aside.

Add mustard, olive oil and white wine vinegar into a little bowl to make the vinaigrette – whisk using a fork until thick and properly mixed.

Remove the pork belly (which is presumably already crispy cooked) from the oven and let it cool. Slice it into fairly small pieces.

Toss the salad greens with your vinaigrette and then top with blue vein cheese, the sliced pork belly, candied nuts and pear.

Save some for dinner.

Nutritional information per serving: Calories: 537.5, Fats 51.46g, Protein 12.74g, Carbs 4.77g

Dinner:

Crispy Pork Salad

Day 10
Breakfast:

Easy Keto Egg Salad

Lunch:

Keto Creamy Meatballs Recipe with Fried Cabbage

Serves 2

Ingredients

<u>For the meatballs</u>

12 ounces ground beef (or ground chicken, ground lamb or ground turkey)

1 egg, whisked

1/2 teaspoon black pepper

2 tablespoons garlic powder

2 teaspoons salt

4 tablespoons coconut oil

<u>The sauce</u>

1/2 medium onion, thinly sliced

2 tablespoons cilantro, chopped

2 tablespoons coconut oil (if required)

Salt and pepper to taste

8 cherry tomatoes, thinly diced

3 cloves of garlic, minced or thinly diced

1/2 cup coconut cream (get this from the top of a chilled coconut milk can)

<u>For the cabbage</u>

1/2 small head of cabbage, thinly shredded

2 tablespoons coconut oil

Salt and pepper to taste

Directions

Mix all the ingredients and shape them properly into balls-each measuring about an inch.

Place a deep pot or pan on high heat and add the four tablespoons of coconut oil; brown the meatballs liberally on all sides. Place them on a plate to rest.

Melt the 2 tablespoons of coconut oil in the same pot (i.e. if you require extra oil); add the onions and fry until browned a bit. Now add the other ingredients for the sauce except the coconut cream.

After five minutes of cooking, you can add the cream. Cook until the cream bubbles and take back the meatballs to the sauce. Simmer, while covered, for 15 minutes.

Now melt two tablespoons of coconut oil when the meatballs are five minutes away from being ready in a big hot pan; throw the cabbage in and fry until it is soft. Season it to your desired taste.

Serve the fried cabbage along with the meatballs in the sauce.

Save some for dinner.

Nutritional information per serving: Calories: 740, Fat 61g, Protein 39g, Carbohydrates 13g

Dinner:

Keto Creamy Meatballs Recipe with Fried Cabbage

Day 11
Breakfast:

Pecan & Cinnamon Porridge

Serves 2

Ingredients

¼ cup of almond butter

¾ cup unsweetened almond milk

2 tablespoon whole chia seeds

¼ cup chopped walnuts or pecans

½ teaspoon cinnamon

¼ cup coconut milk

1 tablespoon extra-virgin coconut oil or MCT oil

2 tablespoon hemp seeds

¼ cup toasted coconut, unsweetened

5-10 drops of liquid stevia or 1-2s tablespoon Erythritol

Directions

Mix the almond milk, coconut milk, coconut oil and almond butter and place over medium high heat to allow it to simmer.

Take off the heat once hot.

Add the hemp seeds, chia seeds, toasted coconut and chopped pecans- you can reserve a bit of coconut for the topping; also add the cinnamon and the stevia if you want. Give it 5-10 minutes to sit after mixing well.

Spoon the porridge into serving bowls then serve cold or hot.

Top with the rest of the coconut just before you serve; enjoy!

Nutritional information per serving: Calories: 580, Fat 51.7g, Protein 13.8g, Carbohydrates 5.2g

Lunch:

Creamy Shrimp And Bacon Skillet

Serves 4

Ingredients

1 pinch Celtic sea salt

4 ounces raw shelled shrimp

1 cup sliced mushrooms

Freshly ground black pepper

½ cup coconut cream or heavy whipping cream

4 ounces smoked salmon

4 slices organic uncured bacon

Instructions

Cut the bacon into bits each measuring one inch.

On a medium high flame, heat a cast iron skillet then place the bacon inside. Cook it while stirring for five or so minutes.

When the bacon cooks, but not yet crispy, add the sliced mushroom and leave it to cook for five minutes. Stir often.

Next, add the shrimp and fry on high for 2 minutes.

Now add the salt cream, decrease the flame and leave it to cook for one minute, or until the cream attains the thickness you want.

Serve with shirataki or zucchini noodles- immediately.

Save some for dinner.

Nutritional information per serving: Calories 340, Fat 29g, Proteins 17g, Carbs 3.5g

Dinner:

Creamy Shrimp And Bacon Skillet

Day 12
Breakfast:

Avocado Toad in the Hole

Lunch:

Easy Keto Lasagna Stuffed Portobellos

Dinner:

Easy Keto Lasagna Stuffed Portobellos

Day 13

Breakfast:

Pecan & Cinnamon Porridge

Lunch:

Skillet Vegetable Sausage With Veggies

Serves 4

Ingredients

3 tablespoon butter or ghee

1 small yellow bell pepper that's cut into chunks

2 minced garlic cloves

1 small zucchini, halved lengthwise; cut into moons

1 little red bell pepper that has been cut into chunks

6 cremini mushrooms, quartered

1/2 teaspoon crushed red pepper flakes

5 sliced chicken sausage links

1 small sweet onion that is cut into chunks

1 medium summer squash that's halved lengthwise

1/2 teaspoon Italian seasoning

Sea salt and black pepper, to taste

Directions

Melt the butter in a large skillet, over medium heat.

Now add the garlic, onion and chicken sausage to the skillet. Sauté for ten minutes.

Add the mushrooms, bell peppers, squash and zucchini, pepper, sea salt, red pepper flakes and Italian seasoning and sauté for 10-15 more minutes, or until the veggies become crisp tender.

Save some for dinner.

Nutritional information per serving: Calories 317, Fats 23g, Protein 20g, Carbohydrates 8g

Dinner:

Skillet Vegetable Sausage With Veggies

Day 14
Breakfast:

Almond Cream Cheese Pancakes

Lunch:

Low carb shepherd's pie

Dinner:

Low Carb Italian Eggs in Purgatory

89

Day 15
Breakfast:

Green Smoothie Bow

Lunch:

Low Carb Italian Eggs in Purgatory

Dinner:

Easy Leftover Turkey Casserole Recipe With Mayonnaise

Day 16
Breakfast:

Cream Cheese Pancakes

Lunch:

Easy Leftover Turkey Casserole Recipe With Mayonnaise

Dinner:

Keto Lasagna with Zucchini Noodles

Day 17
Breakfast:

Easy Keto Egg Salad

Lunch:

Easy Shrimp Avocado Salad With Tomatoes And Feta

Dinner:

Easy Shrimp Avocado Salad With Tomatoes And Feta

Day 18
Breakfast:

Almond Cream Cheese Pancakes

Lunch:

Low Carb Italian Eggs in Purgatory

Dinner:

Keto Sausage and Egg Breakfast Sandwich

Day 19
Breakfast:

Almond Cream Cheese Pancakes

Lunch:

Low Carb Quiche

Dinner:

Low Carb Quiche

Day 20
Breakfast:

Green Smoothie Bow

Lunch:

Crispy Pork Salad

Dinner:

Crispy Pork Salad

Day 21
Breakfast:

Easy Keto Egg Salad

Lunch:

Keto Creamy Meatballs Recipe with Fried Cabbage

Dinner:

Keto Creamy Meatballs Recipe with Fried Cabbage

Day 22
Breakfast:

Pecan & Cinnamon Porridge

Lunch:

Creamy shrimp and bacon skillet

Dinner:

Creamy shrimp and bacon skillet

Day 23
Breakfast:

Avocado toad in the Hole

Lunch:

Easy Keto Lasagna Stuffed Portobellos

Dinner:

Easy Keto Lasagna Stuffed Portobellos

Day 24
Breakfast:

Pecan & Cinnamon Porridge

Lunch:

Skillet Vegetable Sausage With Veggies

Dinner:

Skillet Vegetable Sausage With Veggies

Day 25
Breakfast:

Almond Cream Cheese Pancakes

Lunch:

Low carb shepherd's pie

Dinner:

Low Carb Italian Eggs in Purgatory

Day 26
Breakfast:

Green Smoothie Bow

Lunch:

Low Carb Italian Eggs in Purgatory

Dinner:

Easy Leftover Turkey Casserole Recipe With Mayonnaise

Day 27
Breakfast:

Cream Cheese Pancakes

Lunch:

Easy Leftover Turkey Casserole Recipe With Mayonnaise

Dinner:

Keto Lasagna with Zucchini Noodles

Day 28
Breakfast:

Easy Keto Egg Salad

Lunch:

Easy Shrimp Avocado Salad With Tomatoes And Feta

Dinner:

Easy Shrimp Avocado Salad With Tomatoes And Feta

Day 29
Breakfast:

Almond Cream Cheese Pancakes

Lunch:

Low Carb Italian Eggs in Purgatory

Dinner:

Keto Sausage and Egg Breakfast Sandwich

Day 30
Breakfast:

Green Smoothie Bow

Lunch:

Crispy Pork Salad

Dinner:

Crispy Pork Salad

Conclusion

We have come to the end of the book. Thank you for reading and congratulations for reading until the end.

Well, it's time to do your part. The recipes are simple and few; you will thus be able to learn them quickly before looking for more after the 30th day- which I'd very much encourage.

Enjoy your keto journey to the ultimate good health.

If you found the book valuable, can you recommend it to others? One way to do that is to post a review on Amazon.

Thank you and good luck!

Preview Of 'Ketogenic Cooking: Ketogenic Cooking With Your Instant Pot'

Ketogenic Cooking: Getting Started

The ketogenic diet is a high fat low carb diet designed to allow the body enter a state of ketosis. In this state, your body relies on fat for energy.

Usually, our bodies prefer carbohydrates for energy. Therefore, when you take a high carb meal, the carbohydrates are converted to glucose and the body uses the glucose for energy. Any excess glucose is converted to fat for storage. The more carbohydrates you take, the more any excess are converted to fat for storage. Over time, as your increase your carbohydrate intake, you also increase your fat storage, which only leads to weight gain. With the Ketogenic diet, you reduce your carbohydrate intake, which makes your body look for alternative sources of energy; hence, turning to burning fat for energy.

Adopting the ketogenic diet entails following some rules with regards to the quantities of your macronutrients, which include:

Fats - Fats make the ketogenic diet the success that it is. If you don't consume enough fats, you might as well stop following the diet. This is because you need to get 70% of your daily calories from fat.

Proteins – Get 20% of your daily calories from protein. Avoid eating too much protein since excess proteins can be converted to glucose. This is done via gluconeogenesis. If your protein intake is too much, you risk getting out of ketosis, as your body will have all the glucose it needs and it won't need to burn fat for energy.

Carbohydrates - Carbohydrates have little room in the ketogenic diet. Eat only 50g or 20-25g net carbs each day.

It is important to note that just because you are following the ketogenic diet that your diet will be boring. Actually, this is quite the contrary. Modern appliances and a variety of keto recipes can enable you to enjoy ketogenic recipes for quite some time. One such amazing appliance is the Instant Pot. This top of the range electric pressure cooker comes with several benefits. These include:

Multi-use

You can use the instant pot as a steamer, a sauté pan, a rice cooker and even a slow-cooker. You can also bake in it if you want. If you want to get rid of other appliances and still have various options when cooking, the Instant Pot would be the appliance you'd want to keep. In addition, it doesn't take up a lot of space nor does it heat up the kitchen or make a lot of noise while cooking.

Programmable

We cannot talk about the Instant Pot without mentioning that it is programmable. You can program your Instant Pot 24-hours in advance, if you wish. This function allows you to place your food in the Instant Pot and go about your day without hurrying back to start preparing food. Once it reaches the time you had programmed, your Instant Pot will start doing its work. Thus, by the time you go back home, you'll have a hot freshly cooked meal waiting for you.

Timesaving

The Instant Pot lets you cook meals that would have taken 6-8 hours in a slow cooker in just an hour or even less time. Foods such as a roast can take less than 50 minutes to cook. This gives you more options even if you don't have a lot of time to wait around for meals.

Easy to clean

The Instant Pot makes cleaning easier since its cooking bowl is made of stainless steel; you can easily clean the appliance by hand or place it in the dishwasher. Further, you do not need to scrub it thoroughly. In fact, you should make a habit of cleaning it gently with some soap and warm water. Clean your Instant Pot as soon as you finish cooking. This way, it will be ready when you need to use it again.

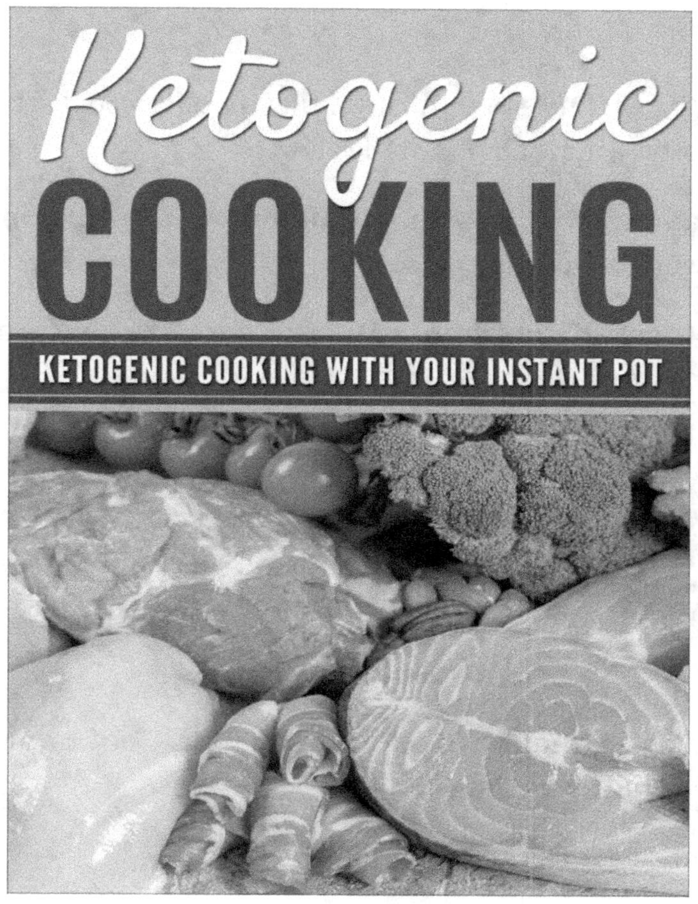

Check out the rest of Ketogenic Cooking on Amazon, go to:
http://amzn.to/2yXp97R

Check Out My Other Books

Below you'll find some of my other popular books that are popular on Amazon and Kindle as well

Alternatively, you can visit my author page on Amazon to see other work done by me.

1. **Ketogenic Cookbook: Quick Low Calorie Ketogenic Crockpot Recipes with 7 Days Meal Plan**

2. **Freedom: How to Make Money Online and Become Financially Free by Creating Passive Income**

3. **Mediterranean Diet: Instant Pot Cookbook with Delicious Recipes**

4. **Alice the Superbug**

5. **Madison and Astrid's first magical journey**

6. Intermittent Fasting: The Essential Beginners Guide for Women for Weight Loss

7. Chakra Healing: Chakra Healing and Karmic Awareness for Beginners

8. SEO 2017 for Growth: The Ultimate Guide to Learn Search Engine Optimization with Internet Marketing Tips

9. Psychology: How to Analyze People Using Human Psychological Techniques, Body Language Signals, Social Skills and Personality Types

10. Paleo Smoothies: Recipes to Energize and for Ultimate Health and Weight Loss

11. Belly Diet Smoothies: Delicious Smoothie Recipes to Flatten Your Belly, Improve Your Gut & Burn Fat

18.Make Money Online To Achieve Freedom

19.Negative Calorie Diet with Smart Fat Guide

20. Negative Calorie Diet & Clean Eating: Cookbook & Guide Which Will Help You To Burn Body Fat, Lose Weight And Live Healthy

21.Smart Fat: Cookbook with Fat Meals Which Help You to Lose Weight, Get Healthy and Improve Brain Function

22. Anti-Inflammatory Diet Guide: The Guide to Reduce Inflammation and Live a Healthy Life Without Pain

23. Essential Oils: The Young Living Book Guide of Natural Remedies for Beginners for Pets, For Dogs

24. Clean Eating: Cookbook and Guide to Restore Your Body's Natural Balance and Eat Healthy

Bonus: Subscribe To The Free Weight Loss Report

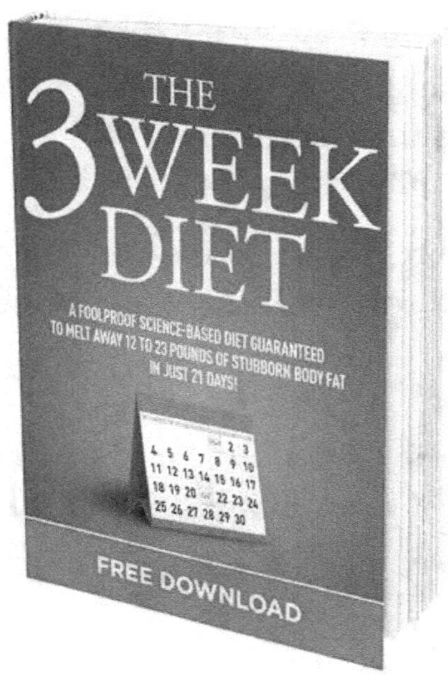

The Introduction Manual is more than just an introduction to the diet. Instead, it discusses the science behind how we gain and lose weight as well as what absolutely needs to be done to attack that stubborn body fat that, until now, has been so challenging to get rid of.

Here are the preview of what you'll get:

- Rapid Weight Loss

- How This System Works

- Why This Diet

- Why 3 Weeks?

- 21 Days To Make A Habit

- Fat Loss VS. Weight Loss

- Nutrients

- Protein, Fat, Carbohydrates

- The Food Pyramid And Obesity

- Fiber

- Metabolism

- How We Get Fat

- Triglycerides

- How To Get Thin

- Diet Overview

- Meal Frequency

- Water

- Diet Essentials

- Let's Get Started

You can access it here: http://bit.ly/2tUb9cp